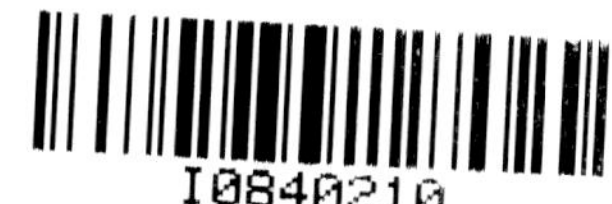

This journal belongs to:

____

Published by Hope Wolf

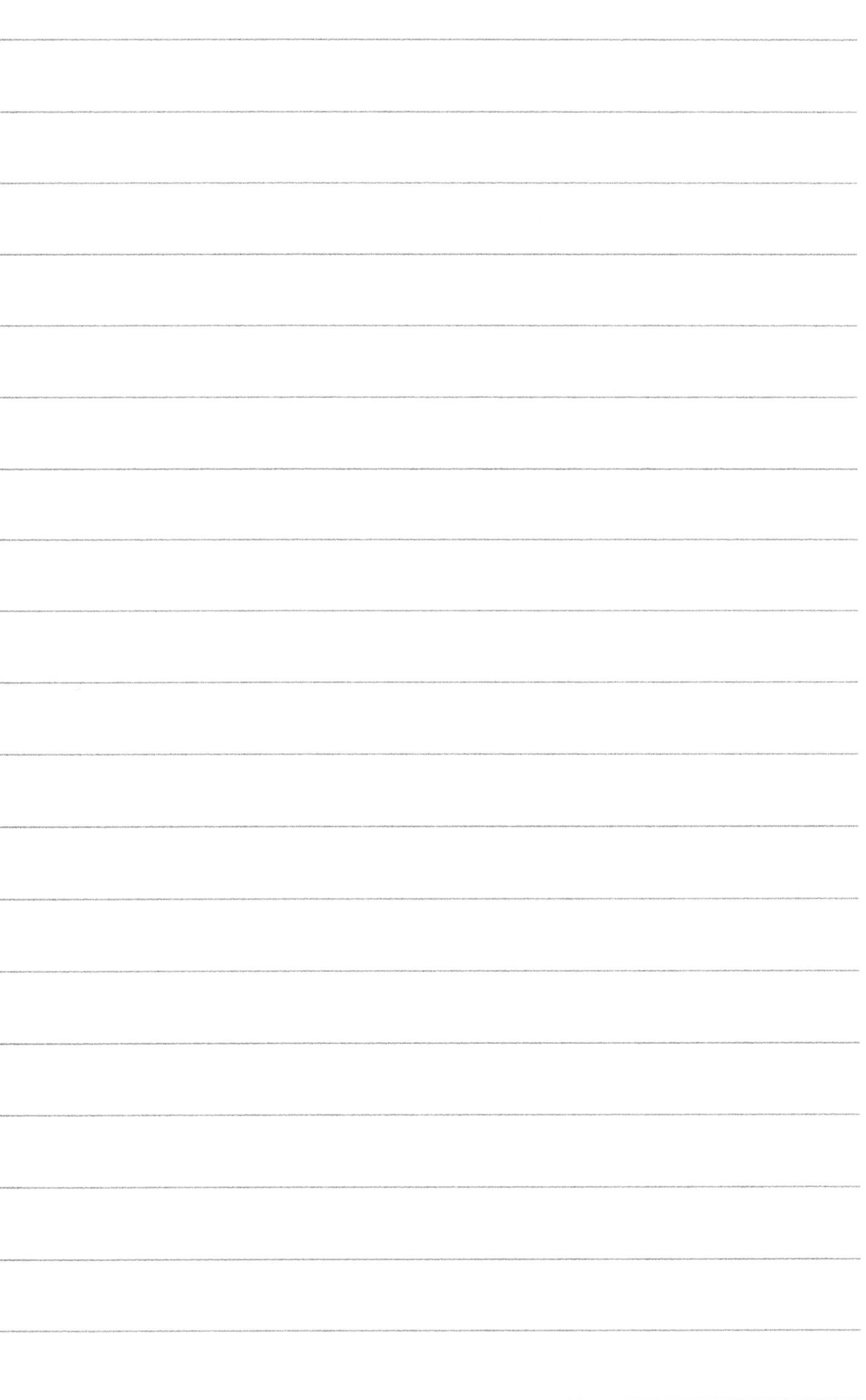

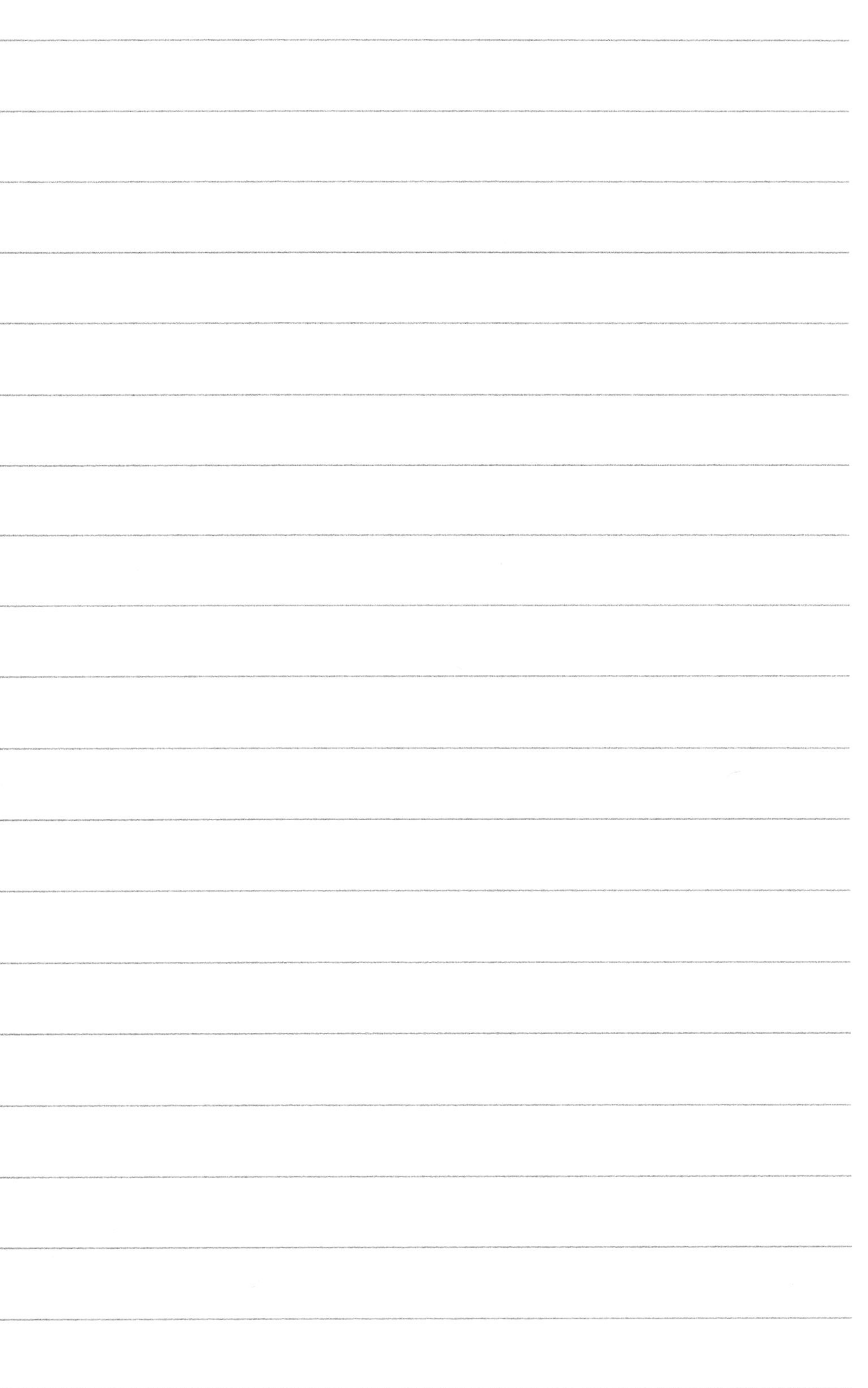

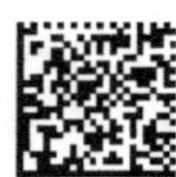